CW01304558

Yoga Poetry

No reproduction without permission

All rights reserved

Copyright © Raj Singh 2009

Yoga Poetry

Yoga Poetry
With Tranquil Minds and Open Hearts

Yoga Poetry

Yoga Poetry

Contents

The Awakening

Great Sky	1
Raise the Curtain	2
Beauty	3
Formation	4
The Gift	5
World Within A World	6
Knot and Bow	7
Pinwheels of Color	8
At Dawn	9
Sunrise	11
Love Poem	12
In The Beginning	13
Morning Storm	15
New Life	16
The First Time	17
Arrival	18

The Pulse of Life

Children	19
The Dance of Discovery	20
Winding River	21
Emerge	22
Resilience	23
Swans	24
Long Line	25
Infinite Rotation	26
Shadow & Light	27
Windmill	28
Palms Together	29
Vines	30

In Thought	31
Drums of the Universe	32
Rainbow	33
Trees	34

The Verve

The Warrior	35
City Sounds	36
Cleaning House	37
Physicality	38
Art of Life	39
Temporary World	40
Upwards	41
Hidden Shadows	43
Call of the Day	44
The Swell	45
Holding the Pose	46
V Formation	47
Jewel	48
Ocean Tide	49
Maintain	51
My Roots	52

Contemplation

In Our Hands	53
Lotus Flower	54
Silent Mind	55
Asana	56
The Breath	57
Grain of Sand	58
Cage	59
Top of the Mountain	60
Consider the Ants	62

Gong Sounds 63
Who Am I? 64
Flowers in the Wind 65
Truth 66
The Seashell 67
Keep It Simple 68
Mind to Body 69

The Afterglow

Just Stars 70
Winter 71
Ascension 72
In Time 73
Beyond Thought 74
Light as Air 76
Eternal Darkness/Eternal Light 77
Sleep Mantra 78
Endless Fire p. 79
Renewal 80
Taper Down 81
The Collective Dream 82
Death Songs 83
Resignation 84
Visions of Spirits 85
Twilight 86

The Awakening

Great Sky

Beneath the canopy of blue

Extending onwards

Rolling outwards to the unknown

On the green blanket

I lay my head,

My hands to my side

Palms open as always

To the great sky

Raise the Curtain

Curtains part to reveal blue sky. Buildings

Allow only a silver, but the light

Prevails, as always. The clouds flicker

In and out of focus, refusing

To dominate the sky

And the sun pokes through the haze,

As the birds begin their chirping, Another

day

Is born -- And I raise the curtain

Beauty

The rays of the sun

Reach even the far corners

Of this Earth

They raise the corn from the ground

And ripen the fruit on the trees

And the rain comes down

To wipe all the slates clean

And there seems no reason for it all,

Unless the reason is simple --

Beauty, existing just to be

Formation

Torn unnaturally it seems

From the safety of the warm insides

Pushed forward without reason

Into uncertainty and fear

Forced to feel the cold

After knowing only warmth

Stark contrasts of black and white

Are what allows life to take form

The Gift

The gift on the table lies un-open

Eyes fall upon it, feel its weight,

Pull at its ribbons

The gift sometimes takes years to open

The young laugh it off

The children ignore it

The gift of life lies on the table,

An unopened box

Few will acknowledge its existence

And fewer still will accept its significance

World Within A World

Hold the morning's breath

Exhale into the night,

Like a world within a world

You are the soul within the flesh

The way you were in lifetimes past

Is present now inside your breath

Knot and Bow

When consciousness shifts,

A veil is lifted

The waves of the day

Bring turmoil and joy,

Together at once

Intricately wrapped

Like two hands laced

Or the knot and bow

Of a ribbon

Pinwheels of Color

From the tip of the tongue to the back of the throat

The inhalation travels down the spine and back out

A tingling sensation fills the frontal lobes,

Bright faces flush red and new sensations are born

The irises spin like pinwheels of color

And the body moves like an eel in the water

New thoughts emerge in bright yellow and blues

And as old thoughts subside, we make room for the new

At Dawn

Beneath the surface

All is stirring

A deep purple hue

Is emerging

Behind the horizon

There is no traffic

Just the birds

Singing,

And the spirit

Waking with each movement

The body stretches

And remembers

As purple becomes orange,

Bursting,

The energy of the day

At dawn

Sunrise

The day begins

With soft rays of light

The wooden beams bend

Beneath the weight of life

With sun salutations, we salute the sun

Our spirit soars & we become one

The sunrise is there

To witness our awakening

Blood and thoughts,

Forever circulating

Warmed by the light, we become calm

Limber and warm, we embrace our true form

Love Poem

We wake together

Move slowly from the bed and

Into downward dog

In the Beginning

In the beginning,

Possibility spreads itself out like wings,

Transcendence looms on the horizon

And the dream is in full swing

The young day is a foal in the beginning

Rising to stand on its own

No one need direct it upwards

For the struggle is nature's true call

In the beginning,

Visions reach heights unimaginable,

The inner eye opens to receive

Our paintings are true to their models

For our work and our art are the same

Morning Storm

Even when the sky is grey, there is beauty

The clouds gently twist and turn, unfurl

Rain a haze of wetness around and through the city

And there within it lies the possibility

Just around the corner, hovering on the horizon,

Through the dampness and the darkness in the sky

A morning storm and a brand new day

New Life

New life will enter the world today

    And the sun will emerge once again

New life will take its first breath today

    As the unknown looms up ahead

Today, a seed will be planted

    And a stalk will sprout from the ground

New life will reach for the stars today

    The world's in the palm of its hand

The First Time

Just as sun repeats it performance,

The world remakes itself every morning

Waterfalls tumble again and again

The birds swoop and play in a compliant wind

From the ground, the trees rise up

As though it was their first time

And the flowers open to reveal colors

As though they has never thought to do so

before

And you walk along the edge of the forest

Listening finally, witnessing it all

As if it was your first time alive in the morning

Arrival

Creatures of the night

Retreat to the underworld

For morning is here

The Pulse of Life

Children

Growing up

We knew how to perch ourselves -

Not like children

Tipping back in our chairs -

But like spotlights

Charring

Black holes in paper,

Illuminating

Severe as the light

Our questions were genuine

Our ideas sparked friction

Like flames in the dark.

The Dance of Discovery

Together in a dance we are the movements

Together we find meaning in this room

Together we see beauty in the ruins

And in the ashes of the fire we see no gloom

Together we move forward through the motions,

Taking each one a moment at a time

Together there will be no secrets

The dance of discovery is for all to see --

We are supporting beams in our prime

Winding River

Know me as I am,

And also as I will be,

For I'm like a river

Winding downstream

I am a transformer

Emerging from the fray

The truth of me emerges

With each passing day

Emerge

After hibernation, comes the stretching

Yawn through your urge to move

There is safety in the dwelling

But no struggle, growth or reward

Emerge from the cave in which you have rested

Sleep was yesterday, now the day is anew

Out here in the wild there are no guarantees

But in the sleep of the fearful there is nothing to see

Resilience

The warm up is the calm

Before the storm of bodies on the street

And the daily onslaught of our duties

The warm up is the building

Of a platform, hammer and nails of the day

The warm up is a secret weapon

A place to jump from, to test the boundaries

Of our mind and our spirit

The warm up is beginning

Of resilience

Swans

The swans hover above the silver

Water, fluffing the silk of their feathers

The wind come and goes, heaves up

And then settles, and the swans remain

Unfazed and free to float, like boats

Just above the silver water

Long Line

The line forms

    Patrons wait

        With expectations

Up ahead,

    Adventure awaits

        But first the long line

Infinite Rotation

Like the phases of the moon passing overhead

The practice fills the space where its most needed

Like the heat of the sun at high noon

The practice warms you from the inside

Like the tide pulling out and returning,

The routine embraces you like an old friend

Just as the rotation of the Earth spins you forward

There is solace in the movements of the wind

Shadow & Light

There is no light without

Shadow

No day without

Night

There's no knowing without

Mystery

No stillness without

Flight

Transformation will restore us

And paupers will be kings

The lost will find their way again

And the silent ones will sing

Windmill

Warm up with spirals

Stretch tall and feel your muscles

The windmill is here

Palms Together

Like the tiny seeds of Springtime

And the buds of newborn stalks

The green innocence inside us

Uproots to carry us forth

With our palms pressed tight together

We trust our hands to find the way

Upwards towards the treetops

We embrace the natural sway

Vines

Inside the young mind --

Intertwined

The vines of thought wrap themselves

Tightly

Ideas grow like ivy --

Making their way upwards

They gain strength from one another

Fast and ever-changing,

Nourished by the joy of life,

Laughter, experience

And love

In Thought

I have been told to control

What I think

For all thoughts eventually

Become words

I have been told to

Control my words

For they can be too fierce

When spoken aloud

And these words can cause you

To act and become

An idea that first existed only

In thought

Drums of the Universe

With the innocence of children

Skipping stones

I exist today

Both hands toward the sky

My feet on the ground

I can sense it

This pulse beating through us

The drums of the universe

May they beat through me, always

Rainbow

The arc of colors,

The world's extension

The ladder to the universe

Beauty within beauty

The combined powers

Of water and sun

The mythology of treasure

A sight to behold

Trees

We should be like trees

Never fighting, just bending

In the autumn wind

The Verve

The Warrior

With hands straight and strong

The warrior pushes through

Intent as an arrow

Aiming for the sun

The warrior stares on

Towards true north

And finds his strength

In the roots of intention

City Sounds

Horns blare

Sirens sounds

The day lurches forward

Find a silent moment

To capture,

To help you maintain

The quiet in your mind

A space in which to hide

From the sounds of the city

Cleaning House

This apartment undulates in the heat,

    With white tiled floors buried under suds

Sweat appears along my brow

    As I wipe at shy corners of dust,

And the dog safe on his throne of laundry

    Watches me; so silly, soaked in sweat

The floor is now sodden.

    And we will wait for it to dry.

Physicality

The body is a vessel

    A physicality waning

A sailboat parting water

    On dry land

It allows our soul to travel,

    Existing purely

In the present-tense

Art of Life

The busy squirrels scamper to and fro

With nuts inside their bulging cheeks

Searching frantically for more

And the tiny birds, whistling in mid-flight

Twist and flit and turn,

Find sticks and leaves to build their home

And watching from my window,

Free from all the strife

I know that I am witnessing

The very art of life

Temporary World

Temporary world

Offers us its shelter

We move through situations

Like Summer into Autumn

But not everything is visible

Like Winter into Spring

There are peaks and darkened valleys

But from each one, we must sing

Upwards

Up & up & up

Stretching, pulling taunt

Muscles working, growing limber

Cells renewing,

Vision clearing,

Thoughts slip away,

The mind releases.

Up & up & up

Balloons lifting, filling

Lungs swelling & receiving

Buoyed upward,

We touch the ceiling,

Then the rooftops,

Then the sky & beyond

Hidden Shadows

In the heat of the day

The shadows will be hiding

But look carefully

Call of the Day

The day calls out for participation

It needs no idle witnesses, but actors

To breathe life into the living

Beneath the sun, the day calls out

For children to play

For all to dance as one

For life to be lived

The day calls out for activity

And from the sidelines we must join

Let's be among the masses,

And let our voices rise in song

The Swell

In the swell,

Time stops

One body,

One mind

One soul,

One heart

The forest parts

The story arcs,

Time stops

In the swell

Holding the Pose

The contraction of the heart

The rise and fall of the chest

In the moment it seems impossible

To continue on without a rest

The teacher stands in front

With a twinkle in her eye

And with the gentlest persuasion

She convinces us to try

To hold the pose a little longer

Count to twenty with each one

And there's nothing quite as nice

As the pleasure of being done

V Formation

Find the rhythm,

Of beating hearts,

Synchronize

The movements

And soar

Like a school of fish

In the sea, uniting

And birds, air born

In V formation

Jewel

Love,

Like a jewel sparkles

Brilliant and unaware

And at the peak of our existence

We might overcome

The glare

Or forget its brilliance

In the spaces in between

And if we miss the mark

And become stranded on the shore

This jewel

Slips through our fingers

Like sand

Lost forever more

Ocean Tide

Like undulations of the tide

I feel the waves within

I never knew I was an ocean

Until my mind began to swim

Everything's alive now

Tingling and aware

Now my is energy peaking

And the day is brightly flared

The sky is much bluer now

The grass, a deeper shade of green

With the yawn of life behind me

I am ready to be seen

Maintain

Every time, the same feeling

Neutrality,

    Then exhilaration,

        Then exhaustion,

            But fleeting

Barely time to catch your breath

Find your strength

And maintain

The pose you've worked

So hard to find

My Roots

My roots are firm and deep

My heart is anew

I'm swaying in the breeze

I've nothing left to hide

I am laughing once again

I am running through the field

I am here now, on this Earth

I am yours to keep

My roots are firm and deep

Contemplation

In Our Hands

In the stillness

Everything has its place

No more spiraling downward

No more fear-based actions

What will be, will be

We can only hold what's in our hands

And I have everything

I need

Lotus Flower

The lotus flower sits

Petals open to the sky

Absorbing all that falls

Snow, soot, sun, rain --

Gifts with purpose

That come and go

The lotus flower lives

In the present time

Patiently alive

Silent Mind

It took awhile to find the silence

It remained a world away for such a time

Now in the aftermath of chaos

I have found my silent mind

It is there to greet me in the morning

And it is there when I feel weak

It has seen a thousand sunsets

But it prefers to listen, not to speak

The silent mind is worth a lifetime

Within it lies the stars and more

If time is how I've found it

Then I wish nothing to be restored

Grain of Sand

Pick a grain of sand

Study it like as you would a close friend

Know the sand,

And know the beach

Know that there is nothing

Too small for contemplation

Cage

Is this a lesson in suffering

Or am I just caught in the storm

Will there be joy on the other side

Or it is destined to pour

These are the questions I ponder

With the weight of the world on my mind

I sit with the best of intentions

With hands opened up to the sky

Waiting for this cage to come open

So at last I can let these thoughts fly

Top of the Mountain

When we were young,

    There were mountains before us,

Looming large in the distance,

    We knew we must climb

We played in their shadow

    Ran through the valleys,

Drank from the streams,

    Thousands of times

At the base of the mountain

    We looked to the top

And now at the summit

    Amidst the wild stillness

There's no more to fear

For the climb is behind us

Consider the Ants

Stop.

Look down.

Consider the ants.

Marching forward.

Where are they going?

Gong Sounds

The gong sounds, slips through our minds like a secret

Vibrations in the floorboards mimic feelings, thoughts

Emotions of the day reverberating, radiating, reaching

Resting. We have come to listen, learn, teach, pray, sing

And be sung to. There are no beginners and no experts,

The gongs sounds, reverberates through our bodies,

Pushing, pulling, breaking, healing. The gong sounds.

Who Am I?

For every being

A different answer

Predicated on actions,

Thoughts and feelings

Who am I?

Why do we live?

Why do we die?

Who should I be?

Who am I?

Flowers in the Wind

`Focus on the quiet,

Let the voices of friends, family, lovers

Bend like flowers in the wind

Focus on the stillness

They are seeds of your enlightenment

From them grow a garden

That will inspire all you know

Truth

The power of Om

The empty and quiet mind

Makes room for the truth

The Seashell

Like the seashell,

    Waiting patiently on the shore,

I will not fight nature's quest

    For balance

And like the seashell,

    I am waiting on eternity

And like the sea shell,

    I will go where I am needed

Keep It Simple

Remember to keep it simple

When you are thirsty, drink

When you are tired, sleep

And if you should find yourself jaded

Focus on the laughter of children

Mind to Body

Out of mind

And into body

There is a force

Burning bright

Within me

Head to toe

Simple and sturdy

Out of mind

And into body

The Afterglow

Just Stars

Not all stories have an ending

Not all rivers lead to the sea

Not all equations have a reason

Not all things are meant to be

Not all information is is worth knowing

Some things just simply are

Only fools insist on answers

When they are staring at the stars

Winter

The winter of life is like phosphorescence

    Radiating from within

The hues deepen and the leaves fall away

    Self and soul become one and the same

Like sleeping and dreaming --

    A blissful forever

Ascension

When the time comes for our ascension

We will rest our busy minds

Our hands will soon fall idle

And we will exhale a heavy sigh

This is not the end,

But a beginning in which we'll find

That the universe has opened

And the eternal embrace is kind

It is here that we reawaken

And our tired eyes will see

That the curtain has been lifted

And we are finally free

In Time

The spirit leaves this world

Like a fire going out

Only to emerge, in time

Stronger and brighter than before

Beyond Thought

Beyond thought

The bells do not ring

The madness continues

Somewhere outside

But here in this room

The world stops

Beyond thought

The birds no not sing

The day begins anew

On the other side of the world

But here in this house

There is silence

The voices are quiet

Beyond thought

The mind floats outward

Beyond thought

Somewhere outside

There is chaos

But here in the mind

The world stops

Light as Air

Finally,

    Silence.

We listen to the sound

    Of nothing.

The buzz gives ways to stillness,

    And our bodies float

On their rafts,

    Light as air,

Light as our breath

    Subsiding,

        Gliding,

            Gently into sleep

Eternal Darkness/Eternal Light

What is this mysterious darkness

That leaves me feeling like a child in the night?

It churns a fear from deep within me

It pulls me from the comfort of my dreams

But I refuse to spend a lifetime hiding from it

Waiting for eternal light to guide me

I must learn the lessons of the darkness

And wait for my fears to turn to joy

For just like waking from a deep and restful slumber

Life and death and two sides of the same coin

Sleep Mantra

Heavy eyes and lids

And the quiet of the night

I will sleep soundly

Endless Fire

In the Heart of your Heart

In the Soul of your Soul

The universe has lit a fire

That forever more will grow

It will never be extinguished

For the seeds of it are pure

And inside this endless fire

Lies the Heart, the Soul and more

Renewal

I used to be afraid of losing control

But I've learned so much since then

My dreams have taught me

To just let go,

Lay down with the earth

And rise anew,

Again and again

Taper Down

Taper down softly

Let the wind be your guide

Not all heights are for jumping off

Travel slow and with pride

Take the longer journey

Remember all you see

Taper down softly

And let the wind set you free

The Collective Dream

Some beds are made of iron

And some are made of straw

Some sleep curled into the corner

Others spread themselves out wide

Some prefer to sleep alone

And others want someone by their side

But all around the world,

No matter how you sleep

We partake in the cycle

And dream the collective dream

Death Songs

Death songs

Sung with joy

From deep in our throats

Through the canyons of life

The sounds we produce

Reverberate wide

The awareness of life

Brings joy to the cycle

And the death songs we sing,

We sing with a smile

Resignation

When I wait in the sunlight

When I take a moment to realize

I am flesh; thin brown hairs on my body;

The scar I call my belly button

Off colored lint floating

In the flood behind my eyes.

When I lay down in the quiet

With shallow breath

And the clouds pass low

Over my head

I realize that this will one day be

A resignation

Visions of Spirits

These visions keep me company,

Grow large behind my eyes

This path must have chosen me,

For everyday I am surprised

As the spirits present themselves

Each night as I lay sleeping

And begin to speak through me

Just when I think I'm dreaming

Twilight

In the twilight of life

We come to a rest,

Stopped in our tracks

Dropped from the whir

Moved from the center

To the periphery

Out of the tornado

And into the air

Printed in Great Britain
by Amazon